BRAIN DIET RECIPES FOR SENIORS

A Quick and Tasty Cookbook for Increasing Cognitive Function, Fighting Alzheimer's and Memory Loss

ANDREW POTTER

TABLE OF CONTENTS

CHAPTER ONE
INTRODUCTION

1.1 Understanding the Importance of Brain Health in Seniors

For seniors, maintaining good brain health is crucial since it has a substantial impact on their general wellbeing and quality of life. Because cognitive ability typically varies with age, maintaining brain health is an essential part of elder care. Comprehending the significance of maintaining cognitive capacities highlights the need for customised strategies, encompassing an emphasis on diet, way of life, and mental stimulation.

Cognitive talents including memory, processing speed, and problem-solving ability might deteriorate as people age. These modifications may affect independence and day-to-day activities. In order to reduce cognitive decline and improve cognitive resilience in the face of ageing, maintaining brain health becomes a proactive strategy.

Seniors' mental health is greatly supported by their diet. A number of nutrients, including vitamins, antioxidants, and omega-3 fatty acids, have been related to cognitive performance and may help avoid neurodegenerative illnesses. A diet high in these nutrients can help maintain synaptic plasticity and lower oxidative stress, which will help the ageing brain function better.

Moreover, emotional stability and mental wellness are enhanced by a healthy brain. Seniors who have cognitive impairment are frequently more likely to experience anxiety and sadness. Seniors who prioritise their mental health via healthy eating and lifestyle choices report higher moods and greater emotional resilience, which contributes to a more contented and meaningful existence.

Maintaining cognitive capacities requires not just nutritional changes but also mental and social engagement. Playing games, picking up new skills, and interacting with others are examples of brain-stimulating activities that might support resilience and cognitive reserve.

In summary, comprehending the importance of brain health in older adults involves more than just acknowledging the cognitive alterations brought on by ageing. It entails realising the significant influence a functioning brain has on one's general well-being, level of independence, and emotional stability. Seniors can experience a more happy and active existence as they age by adopting a holistic strategy that includes mental stimulation, diet, and social interaction.

1.2 How Nutrition Impacts Cognitive Function

The makeup of a person's food and the presence or absence of particular nutrients can have an impact on brain function. Nutrition has a major effect on cognitive performance. those low in simple sugars are linked to issues with focus and attention, whereas those high in glycemic index have been reported to enhance attention, memory, and functional ability. A constant supply of amino acids is needed by the brain to synthesise neurotransmitters, particularly catecholamines and serotonin, which are involved in memory, learning, and thinking. The kind and quality of dietary fat can also have an impact on cognitive function; a high intake of saturated fat is linked to cognitive decline, whereas a diet high in polyunsaturated fatty acids is advantageous in preventing cognitive decline.

Research indicates that a nutritious diet and its constituent parts can help to improve cognitive abilities in general. Certain cognitive domains, including memory and processing speed, are significantly impacted by dietary patterns and individual nutrients. On the other hand, a diet heavy in refined carbohydrates and saturated fats and low in fruits, vegetables, and water can have a detrimental effect on cognitive function. As a result, healthy eating is essential for maintaining cognitive function and maximising brain performance. Early nutritional therapies may be able to avoid cognitive deficiencies caused by early-life diet and stress exposure, which can cause cognitive dysfunction throughout one's life. Taken as a whole, these findings demonstrate the significance of food composition for long-term effects beyond metabolism and point to the encouraging possibility that modest dietary changes might enhance our cognitive abilities far into old age.

CHAPTER TWO
ESSENTIAL NUTRIENTS FOR
BRAIN HEALTH

2.1 Omega-3 Fatty Acids

Essential polyunsaturated fats, omega-3 fatty acids, are critical for maintaining many facets of health, including cardiovascular and brain function. Alpha-linolenic acid (ALA), docosahexaenoic acid (DHA), and eicosapentaenoic acid (EPA) are the three primary forms of omega-3 fatty acids.

The main sources of EPA and DHA are fatty fish like sardines, mackerel, and salmon. These long-chain omega-3 fatty acids have a critical role in neurotransmitter signalling, synaptic plasticity, and the integrity and functionality of brain cell membranes. Sufficient EPA and DHA levels have been linked in studies to a lower incidence of neurodegenerative illnesses and cognitive impairment.

Conversely, plant-based sources of ALA include walnuts, chia seeds, and flaxseeds. Although ALA is also advantageous, it has to be converted by the body into EPA and DHA, which is frequently an ineffective procedure. For this reason, adding marine sources of omega-3s is very crucial for directly acquiring these vital fatty acids.

Omega-3 fatty acids are well known for their cardiovascular advantages in addition to their effects on brain function. They support general heart health by lowering blood triglyceride levels and reducing inflammation. Furthermore, omega-3s may contribute to mental health and have been linked to elevated mood.

A smart dietary decision for general health and longevity is to include omega-3 fatty acids in one's diet from a range of sources, since they have several health advantages, including supporting heart health, cognitive function, and emotional well-being.

2.2 Antioxidants

Antioxidants are substances that are vital in defending the cells of the body from oxidative stress brought on by free radicals. Free radicals are unstable chemicals that are naturally formed as a consequence of metabolism. They may cause damage to cells, including brain cells, and are linked to a number of disorders and the ageing process.

Vitamins C and E, minerals zinc and selenium, and phytochemicals included in fruits, vegetables, and other plant-based diets are examples of common antioxidants. Antioxidants are abundant in leafy greens, almonds, citrus fruits, and berries.

Antioxidants aid in the neutralisation of free radicals, reducing brain cell damage in the context of brain health. This protective effect is essential for maintaining cognitive function and may help reduce the development of neurodegenerative diseases such as Alzheimer's.

Because antioxidants lower inflammation in the body, they also promote general health. Chronic inflammation can have a detrimental effect on cognitive function and is associated with a number of disorders, including cardiovascular problems. Antioxidants provide a healthy environment for the brain to operate in by reducing inflammation.

Antioxidants can be naturally obtained from a diet high in fruits and vegetables, but supplements are also occasionally taken into consideration, particularly for people with certain health issues or deficits. To take advantage of the synergistic benefits of the many chemicals found in whole foods, it is typically advised to receive antioxidants through a diverse and nutrient-dense diet and whole foods.

In conclusion, antioxidants are critical for preserving the integrity of cells, shielding the brain from oxidative stress, and promoting general wellbeing. A practical and pleasurable strategy to support a robust and healthy body, including the brain, is to include a colourful assortment of fruits, vegetables, and other foods high in antioxidants in the diet.

2.3 Vitamins and Minerals

Micronutrients like vitamins and minerals are needed by the body in lesser amounts, yet they are essential for many physiological processes that promote general health and wellbeing. These substances are necessary for healthy development, growth, and preservation of the best possible functioning of the body.

Vitamins:

1. **Vitamin A:** vital for healthy skin, eyesight, and immune system. present in leafy greens, sweet potatoes, and carrots.

2. **The vitamin B complex consists of the following:** B1 (thiamine), B2 (riboflavin), B3

(niacin), B6 (pyridoxine), B9 (folate), and B12 (cobalamin). These vitamins are essential for the synthesis of red blood cells, neuron function, and energy metabolism. Leafy greens, meat, dairy, and whole grains are some of the sources.

3. **Vitamin C:** An effective antioxidant that promotes collagen formation and the immune system. present in bell peppers, strawberries, and citrus fruits.

4. **Vitamin D:** Essential for calcium absorption and the health of bones. Sources include fatty fish, sun exposure, and fortified dairy products.

5. **Vitamin E:** a potent antioxidant that protects cells from harm. present in seeds, nuts, and vegetable oils.

6. **Vitamin K:** Essential for blood clotting and bone health. Leafy greens, broccoli, and soybean oil are good sources.

Minerals:

1. **Calcium:** vital for maintaining healthy bones and teeth, neurological function, and muscular tone. Calcium may be found in dairy products, leafy greens, and fortified meals.

2. **Iron:** Required for the blood to carry oxygen. present in beans, red meat, and fortified grains.

3. Magnesium: Promotes bone health, muscle and neurological function. Rich in magnesium include leafy greens, nuts, and seeds.

4. **Potassium:** Essential for preserving fluid balance and heart health. Citrus fruits, potatoes, and bananas are good sources.

5. **Zinc:** Promotes wound healing and immunological function. present in dairy, legumes, and meat.

Ensuring an appropriate intake of vitamins and minerals is facilitated by a diverse and balanced diet that encompasses a range of fruits, vegetables, whole grains, and lean meats. This, in turn, promotes general health and vigour.

CHAPTER THREE
BREAKFAST BOOSTERS
3.1 Blueberry Walnut Smoothie

Satisfy your palate and feed your mind with this colourful smoothie that combines the best of both worlds—freshness and nutty deliciousness. This smoothie provides a nutritional boost for your cognitive health in addition to being a tasty treat for your taste buds since it is loaded with antioxidants, omega-3 fatty acids, and important vitamins.

Ingredients:
- 1-ripe banana
- 1 cup blueberries, either fresh or frozen
- Half a cup of yoghurt
- 1/4 cup of walnuts, chopped
- One-third cup chia seeds
- One cup almond milk (or any other type of milk).
- Ice cubes, if desired

Instructions:

1. **Prepare the Ingredients:**
   - Thoroughly wash the blueberries.
   - For easier mixing, peel the ripe banana and cut it into smaller parts.
   - Measure out the chia seeds, chopped walnuts, and Greek yoghurt.

2. **Combine in Blender:**
   - Place the blueberries, Greek yoghurt, chopped walnuts, banana chunks, and chia seeds in a blender.
   - Add the almond milk until the mixture blends well.
   - Add a few ice cubes to the smoothie if you would like it cooler.

3. **Blend Until Smooth:**
   - Tighten the blender's cover and process the components until a silky-smooth consistency is reached.
   - Every now and then stop to scrape down the edges to ensure equal mixing.

4. **Serve and Savour:**
   - Transfer the decadent blend into a glass or your preferred smoothie cup.

- Garnish with a few whole blueberries or a sprinkle of chopped walnuts for an extra touch.

5. Savor the Nutrient-Rich Refreshment:
- Savour the cool flavour of blueberries combined with a hint of crunch from the walnuts.
- Savour the knowing that every drink enhances the health of your brain since it contains powerful antioxidants and omega-3 fatty acids.

This smoothie with blueberries and walnuts is not only a delicious treat, but it's also a nutritious powerhouse that will boost your brain health and give your day a taste boost. Drink, taste, and feed your brain with each delicious sip.

3.2 Avocado and Spinach Omelette

Take a trip through taste and nutrition with the Avocado and Spinach Omelette, a morning wonderland that blends the brilliant freshness of spinach with the creamy richness of avocado. In addition to tantalising your taste senses, this straightforward yet decadent meal gives you a healthy dose of vital nutrients to start the day off right.

Ingredients:
- Two big eggs
- Half a ripe avocado, sliced;
- One tablespoon olive oil;
- A handful of freshly cut spinach leaves; salt and pepper to taste;
- Additional toppings, such as diced tomatoes, feta cheese, or a sprinkling of fresh herbs

Instructions:
1. Prepare the Ingredients:
- After cracking the eggs into a bowl, thoroughly whisk them together.
- Cut up the fresh spinach leaves and slice the avocado.

2. Heat the Pan:
- Set a nonstick skillet over medium heat and drizzle with olive oil. Let the pan become hot.

3. **Cook the Spinach:**
   - Add the chopped spinach and sauté it in the hot pan until it wilts. It should take one or two minutes to complete.
4. **Add the Whisked Eggs:**
   - Ensure that the spinach is evenly distributed throughout the pan of sautéed spinach by pouring the whisked eggs over it.
5. **Add Avocado Slices:**
   - Top one side of the omelette with the avocado slices. When folded, this guarantees the ideal combination of flavours.
6. **Season and Fold:**
   - Sprinkle salt and pepper over the eggs and let them cook until the edges start to set.
   - Carefully fold the omelette in half, covering the avocado and creating a delightful pocket of goodness.
7. **Cook to Perfection:**
   - Continue cooking until the eggs are fully set but still moist, adjusting heat as needed.

8. **Garnish and Serve:**
   - Optionally, add diced tomatoes, feta cheese, or fresh herbs as a finishing touch.
   - Slide the omelette onto a plate, ready to be enjoyed.

The powerful combination of avocado and spinach in this omelette not only boosts nutrition but also pleases the mouth with its rich, creamy texture. With this nutritious and tasty breakfast alternative, you can kickstart your morning while satisfying your hunger and your body.

3.3 Chia Seed Pudding with Berries

Savour a guilt-free dessert that is good for your health and your taste buds: Chia Seed Pudding with Berries. Simple chia seeds are elevated to a velvety, gratifying pudding with the added sweetness of berries in this quick and simple dish. This meal is a healthy way to add vital nutrients to your diet, whether it is eaten as a dessert or as a filling breakfast.

Ingredients:
- Half a cup of chia seeds
- One cup of milk (dairy, almond, or coconut)
- One tablespoon honey or maple syrup, adjusted to taste
- A half-teaspoon of vanilla essence
- A mixture of raspberries, blueberries, and strawberries to garnish

Instructions:

1. Combine Chia Seeds and Liquid:
- Place the chia seeds in a dish and add your preferred milk, making sure the seeds are fully soaked. In order to prevent clumping, stir well.

2. Add Sweetener and Flavour:
- To add sweetness, use honey or maple syrup.
- To enhance flavour, add a small amount of vanilla essence. To suit your tastes, adjust the sweetness.

3. **Stir and Chill:**
   - Give the mixture another stir, put the bowl lid on, and chill it for two or more hours or overnight.
   - The liquid will be absorbed by the chia seeds, giving the mixture a pudding-like consistency.

4. **Inspect and Mix Once More:**
   - Examine the custard following the first chilling time.
   - To get the right consistency, mix in a little milk if it's too thick.

5. **Assemble with Berries:**
   - Spoon the custard into serving dishes or glasses after it reaches the correct thickness.
   - Scatter a vibrant selection of mixed berries over the custard.

6. **Present and Savour:**
   - It's time to enjoy this Chia Seed Pudding with Berries.
   - A beautiful symphony of flavours and textures is produced when the burst of

freshness from the berries is combined with the creamy chia pudding.

7. **Optional Garnishes:**
   - You may add a few mint leaves, crushed coconut, or a drop of honey as an added touch.

This dish gives you a healthy dose of omega-3 fatty acids, fibre, and antioxidants from the chia seeds and berries, in addition to satisfying your sweet tooth. Savour this adaptable delicacy guilt-free, knowing that every spoonful enhances your general wellbeing and your sense of taste.

CHAPTER FOUR
LUNCH FOR COGNITIVE FUNCTION

4.1 Salmon Salad with Mixed Greens

Upgrade your meal experience with a salmon salad that has a colourful combination of greens. This salad, which blends the richness of salmon with the crisp freshness of various greens, is full of flavour and nutrients. It will take your taste senses on a delightful journey while also providing a nutritious boost to your general well-being.

Ingredients:

- One pound of baked or grilled salmon fillets
- One cup of halved cherry tomatoes;
- six cups of mixed salad greens (arugula, spinach and romaine)
- One cucumber, sliced
- One diced avocado
- Half a red onion, finely sliced
- Fresh dill to decorate

For the Dressing:
- 3 tablespoons olive oil
- 2 tablespoons balsamic vinegar
- 1 teaspoon Dijon mustard
- Salt and pepper to taste

Instructions:

1. **Prepare the Salmon:**
   - The salmon fillets should be cooked to perfection on a grill or baking sheet. Let them cool somewhat and then break them into little pieces.

2. **Assemble the Greens:**
   - Put the chopped avocado, cucumber slices, halved cherry tomatoes, red onion slices, and mixed greens into a big salad bowl.

3. **Add Flaked Salmon:**
   - Evenly scatter the flaked salmon over the mixed greens, ensuring that the textures and flavours are well-balanced.

4. **Whisk the Dressing:**
   - In a small bowl, mix together the olive oil, balsamic vinegar, Dijon mustard, salt, and pepper. This gives the salad dressing a tart and harmonious flavour.

5. **Drizzle and Toss:**
   - Pour the dressing over the salad and gently toss to cover every component with an equal layer of the delicious dressing.

6. **Garnish with Fresh Dill:**
   - To give a last flourish of herbal flavour, sprinkle some fresh dill over the salad.

7. **Present and Savour:**
   - Arrange the Salmon Salad on a platter with Mixed Greens, forming a visually appealing composition of hues and textures.
   - A healthy and filling dinner is produced when juicy salmon, crisp greens, and a spicy dressing are combined.

8. **Optional give-ons:**
   - To give a bit more crunch and flavour, try crumbled feta cheese or roasted almonds.

With its delicious combination of ingredients, this salmon salad not only pleases the palate but also has several health advantages. This salad, loaded with proteins, vitamins, and minerals, is a perfect example of how to balance taste buds with health. It's also high in omega-3 fatty acids.

4.2 Quinoa and Vegetable Buddha Bowl

The Quinoa and Vegetable Buddha Bowl is a colourful, nutrient-dense dish that offers a symphony of textures and flavours. Dive into a world of nutrients and flavours with this dish. In addition to being a visual feast, this Buddha Bowl celebrates healthful foods by blending quinoa, vibrant veggies, and an enticing sauce to create a gastronomic beauty.

Ingredients:
- 1 cup quinoa, rinsed and cooked
- 1 cup broccoli florets, steamed
- 1 cup cherry tomatoes, halved
- 1 medium carrot, julienned
- 1/2 cucumber, sliced
- 1/2 avocado, sliced
- 1/4 cup hummus
- Sesame seeds and fresh cilantro for garnish

For the Tahini Dressing:
- 3 tablespoons tahini
- 2 tablespoons lemon juice
- 1 tablespoon olive oil
- 1 clove garlic, minced
- Salt and pepper to taste
- Water to adjust consistency

Instructions:
1. Cook Quinoa:

- After giving the quinoa a quick rinse in cold water, cook it as directed on the package. Using a fork, fluff and allow to cool somewhat.

2. **Get the veggies ready.**
   - Broccoli florets should be steamed until crisp-tender.
   - Slices of avocado, cucumber, cherry tomatoes, and julienned carrot should be ready.

3. **Assemble the Buddha Bowl:**
   - To create an eye-catching appearance, divide the quinoa, steamed broccoli, cherry tomatoes, julienned carrot, cucumber slices, and avocado slices into parts in a bowl.

4. **Add Hummus:**
   - To add a creamy and savoury touch to the bowl, spoon hummus into the centre or on the side.

5. **Make Tahini Dressing:**
   - Mix the tahini, lemon juice, olive oil, minced garlic, salt, and pepper in a small

bowl. Use water to adjust the consistency until the required thickness is reached.

6. **Drizzle Dressing and Garnish:**
   - On top of the Quinoa and Vegetable Buddha Bowl, drizzle the tahini dressing.
   - For a last pop of flavour and texture, add some sesame seeds and fresh cilantro.
7. **Present and Savour:**
   - Slurp up this nutrient-dense bowl, making sure every mouthful is a tasty blend of grains, veggies, and the creamy tahini sauce.
8. **Customise as desired:**
   - You are welcome to add more toppings to the bowl, such as nuts, seeds, or your preferred source of protein.

This Quinoa and Vegetable Buddha Bowl is more than just a dish; it's a whole experience that delights your senses with a wide variety of flavours and textures while providing your body with vital nutrients. Accept the elegance of a well-rounded, healthful food that combines culinary skill with dietary knowledge.

4.3 Tomato Basil Soup with Whole Grain Crackers

Take a trip to a gourmet paradise with the flavorful Basil Soup and the nutritious crunch of Whole Grain Crackers. This dish is delicious because it has a hint of spice from the basil and the hearty richness of whole grain crackers combined with the cosy warmth of a well-made soup.

Ingredients:
- 2 cups fresh basil leaves, packed
- 2 tablespoons olive oil
- 1 onion, diced
- 2 cloves garlic, minced
- 4 cups vegetable or chicken broth
- 4 large tomatoes, diced
- Salt and pepper to taste
- 1/2 cup heavy cream (optional)
- Whole grain crackers for serving

Instructions:

1. **Sauté Aromatics:**
   - Warm up the olive oil in a big saucepan over medium heat. Sauté diced onions until translucent, then add minced garlic and cook until fragrant.

2. **Add Basil and Tomatoes:**
   - Stir in the fresh basil leaves, allowing them to wilt and release their aromatic essence.
   - Add diced tomatoes to the pot, letting them soften and infuse the soup with their natural sweetness.

3. **Simmer the Soup:**
   - Add the chicken or vegetable broth and boil the mixture until it becomes slightly tender. Give the flavours a good fifteen to twenty minutes to mingle and merge.

4. **Perfectly Season:**

- Add salt and pepper to taste while seasoning the soup. Tailor the seasoning to your personal taste.

5. **Mix for Smoothness:**
- Use an immersion blender to carefully mix the soup until it's smooth, for a velvety texture. Or, transfer the soup to a blender in batches.

6. **Optional Creaminess:**
- If you'd like, mix in heavy cream for extra richness. Although optional, this step helps create a rich, creamy finish.

7. **Get Ready for Whole Grain Crackers:**
- Arrange the crackers on a tray for presentation. These crackers not only add a satisfying crunch but also bring a dose of whole grains to the meal.

8. **Serve and Enjoy:**
- Pour the Basil Soup into individual bowls and, if preferred, top with more basil leaves.

- Serve each dish with a side of whole grain crackers to provide a fun tactile contrast.

9. **Appreciate the Harmony**

- Enjoy the pleasant crunch of whole grain crackers and the aromatic, flavorful soup as you revel in the harmony of flavours.

The skill of balance in culinary creations is demonstrated by this Basil Soup with Whole Grain Crackers. It combines the satisfying crunch of whole grains with the fragrant freshness of basil to create a meal that not only pleases the palate but also nourishes it with the health of whole foods. Savour the comforting warmth of this delicious soup, which goes well with the nutritious crunch of whole grain crackers.

CHAPTER FIVE
SNACK TIME BRAIN BITES

5.1 Trail Mix with Nuts and Dried Fruits

Make your own Trail Mix, a delicious and nutritious snack that will satisfy your need for nuts and dried fruits, to start your road towards a more savoury, high-energy lifestyle. Not only is this adaptable blend tasty, but it's also a healthy and practical choice for an instant energy boost.

Ingredients:
- 1 cup almonds
- 1 cup walnuts
- 1/2 cup cashews
- 1/2 cup pumpkin seeds
- 1/2 cup dried cranberries
- 1/2 cup raisins
- 1/2 cup dried apricots, chopped
- 1/4 cup dark chocolate chips (optional)
- 1/4 teaspoon sea salt (optional)

Instructions:

1. **Select Quality Ingredients:**
   - Selecting premium nuts and dried fruits will maximise flavour and nutritional value.

2. **Prepare the Nuts:**
   - Roasting the raw nuts will bring out their flavour. In a dry skillet set over medium heat, roast the nuts, tossing often, until aromatic and brown.
   - Give them time to cool.

3. **Mix Nuts and Dried Fruits:**
   - Put almonds, walnuts, cashews, pumpkin seeds, raisins, dried cranberries, and chopped dried apricots in a big dish.
   - To equally spread the ingredients, thoroughly mix.

4. **Optional Chocolate Indulgence:**
   - You can add dark chocolate chips to the mixture if you'd like a little sweetness.

- The natural richness of the fruits is complemented by the slight bitterness of the dark chocolate.

5. **Sprinkle with Sea Salt (Optional):**
   - Sprinkle a small amount of sea salt on top of the trail mix for a savoury edge. This brings out the flavours and creates a lovely contrast.
6. **Toss for Even Distribution:**
   - Combine the ingredients, making sure that the nuts, fruits, and any extra additions are distributed evenly.
7. **Portion into Snack Packs:**
   - For convenient access throughout the week, divide the trail mix into smaller amounts or keep it in an airtight container.
8. **Savour on the Go:**
   - Whether you're hiking, at work, or just generally on the go, grab a handful of our wholesome Trail Mix anytime you need a fast energy boost.
9. **Tailor to Your Taste:**

- To add even more nourishment, try experimenting with other nuts, dried fruits, or even seeds like flax or chia.

Not simply a snack, this Trail Mix with Nuts and Dried Fruits is a tasty blend of textures and flavours that provides your body with vital nutrients. Whether you lead a hectic lifestyle or are an explorer, our handmade trail mix offers a delightful and practical way to keep your energy levels up all day.

5.2 Greek Yogurt Parfait with Granola

Take your taste buds on a delightful culinary adventure by making a Greek yoghurt parfait with healthy granola on top. This harmonious blend of flavours and textures turns breakfast or snack time into a moment of pleasure and nourishment. This easy-to-make yet incredibly delicious parfait blends the natural sweetness of fresh fruit with the crunchy granola and creamy richness of Greek yoghurt.

Ingredients:

- 1 cup Greek yogurt
- 1/2 cup granola (store-bought or homemade)
- 1 tablespoon honey or maple syrup
- Fresh berries (strawberries, blueberries, raspberries)
- Sliced bananas or other fruits of choice
- Chopped nuts (optional)

Instructions:

1. **Choose Quality Ingredients:**
   - Pick a premium Greek yoghurt that is best enjoyed unsweetened so that the flavours may come through naturally.

2. **Layer Greek Yoghurt:**
   - To start, add a layer of Greek yoghurt to the bottom of a glass or bowl to give your parfait a creamy base.

3. **Drizzle with Honey or Maple Syrup:**
   - To give a hint of natural sweetness, drizzle honey or maple syrup over the yoghurt layer.
   - Adapt the quantity to your personal taste.

4. **Add a coating of Granola:**

- Cover the yoghurt with a thick coating of granola. The granola offers a satisfying crunch and a substantial serving of nutritious grains.

5. **Top with Fresh Fruits:**
   - To add a pop of colour and natural sweetness, top with a layer of fresh berries like raspberries, strawberries, or blueberries. Intersperse with sliced bananas or your favorite fruits.

6. **Repeat for a Beautiful Parfait:**
   - Repeat the layering process until you reach the top of the glass or bowl, creating a visually appealing parfait with alternating layers of yogurt, granola, and fresh fruits.

7. **Top with Nuts (Optional):**
   - Sprinkle chopped nuts (almonds or walnuts) on top for a little crunch and a boost of good fats.

8. **Serve right away and enjoy:**
   - Savour the harmonic fusion of crunchy granola, creamy yoghurt, and the inherent richness of fresh fruit by digging into this

delicious Greek Yoghurt Parfait with Granola right away.

9. **Tailor to Your Taste:**
   - You are welcome to add more toppings to the parfait, including shredded coconut, chia seeds, or a dollop of nut butter.

This Greek Yoghurt Parfait with Granola is more than simply a meal; it's a feast for the senses, elevating a basic yoghurt snack to a wonderful and fulfilling experience. This parfait, whether eaten for breakfast or as a filling snack, is a beautiful example of how to blend crunchy and creamy ingredients together harmoniously.

5.3 Dark Chocolate Covered Almonds

Enjoy a delectable combination of crunchy almonds covered in a rich coating of dark chocolate that will elevate your snacking experience. These are called Dark Chocolate Covered Almonds. This simple-to-make treat gives a dose of heart-healthy almonds and the antioxidant-rich richness of dark chocolate in addition to satisfying your sweet tooth.

Ingredients:
- 1 cup raw almonds
- 1 cup dark chocolate chips or chopped dark chocolate
- 1 tablespoon coconut oil
- 1/2 teaspoon vanilla extract
- Sea salt for sprinkling (optional)

Instructions:
1. **Prepare Almonds:**
   - In a pan over medium heat, dry-roast the raw almonds, turning often, until golden brown and fragrant with nuts. This procedure improves the flavour of the almonds.
2. **Melt Dark Chocolate:**
   - Use a double boiler or brief microwave bursts to melt chopped dark chocolate or dark chocolate chips in a heatproof basin.

- Add coconut oil and stir to get a glossy, smooth consistency.

3. **Add Vanilla essence:**
   - To add even more flavour to the chocolate, incorporate a small amount of vanilla essence into the melted mixture.

4. **Coat Almonds:**
   - Add the roasted almonds to the bowl once the chocolate has melted and been thoroughly combined. Make sure all the almonds are well covered with the rich chocolate.

5. **Arrange on Parchment Paper:**
   - Use parchment paper to line a baking sheet. Make sure the chocolate-covered almonds are not clumped together by arranging them in a single layer.

6. **Cool and Set:**
   - You may speed up this process by putting the baking sheet in the refrigerator for approximately half an hour, or you can let

the chocolate-covered almonds cool and set at room temperature.

7. **Top with Sea Salt (Optional):**
   - While the chocolate-covered almonds are still a little sticky, top them with a little teaspoon of sea salt for a gourmet touch. The salt creates a lovely contrast and brings out the sweetness.

8. **Break Into Clusters:**
   - After the almonds have completely hardened, break them into clusters or separate pieces. The outcome is a delectable arrangement of almond pleasures wrapped in dark chocolate.

9. **Store and Enjoy:**
   - The Dark Chocolate Covered Almonds should be kept cold and closed in a container. Savour these rich candies as a beautiful handcrafted present or as a filling snack.

10. **Experiment with Variations:**

- Feel free to try adding a little of chilli powder for a spicy kick, or even just a sprinkling of cocoa powder or cinnamon.

The nutty crunch of almonds combined with the velvety richness of dark chocolate creates a magical combination that is demonstrated in this recipe for Dark Chocolate Covered Almonds. Satisfy your sweet desire while gaining from dark chocolate's antioxidants and almonds' nutritional advantages. These handcrafted treats are sure to become a treasured pleasure, whether they are enjoyed alone or with others.

CHAPTER SIX
DINNER DELIGHTS FOR THE MIND
6.1 Baked Salmon with Lemon and Herbs

Enjoy a more sophisticated and refined meal with Baked Salmon that has been infused with the fragrant fragrance of herbs and the zesty brightness of lemon. With each bite, this dish produces a symphony of flavours that dance on your palette, showcasing the inherent richness of salmon. As a consequence, you have a dish that celebrates the harmony of using high-quality, fresh ingredients while still tasting excellent.

Ingredients:
- 4 salmon fillets, skin-on.
- 1 lemon, thinly sliced
- 2 tablespoons fresh lemon juice
- 3 tablespoons olive oil
- 2 cloves garlic, minced
- 1 tablespoon fresh dill, chopped
- 1 tablespoon fresh parsley, chopped
- Salt and pepper to taste

Instructions:

1. **Preheat the Oven:**
   - Preheat your oven to 375°F (190°C). This ensures a consistent and even bake for the salmon.

2. **Prepare the Salmon Fillets:**
   - Pat the salmon fillets dry with paper towels. This helps achieve a crisp exterior during baking.

3. **Season with Herbs and Spices:**
   - Combine the minced garlic, chopped parsley, chopped dill, olive oil, fresh lemon juice, salt, and pepper in a small bowl. This gives the fish a tasty marinate.

4. **Marinate the Salmon:**
   - Place the skin-side down salmon fillets on a baking tray. Make sure the flavours of the herb and lemon mixture get into the salmon by liberally coating each fillet.

5. **Add Lemon Slices to the Top:**
   - Top each fillet with a circle of thinly sliced lemon. The lemon gives the salmon

a refreshing taste and a visually pleasing accent at the same time.

6. **Bake to Perfection:**
   - Bake the salmon for about 15 to 20 minutes, or until a fork can easily pierce it, in the preheated oven. The cooking time may be different depending on the thickness of the fillets.

7. **Broil for a Crisp Finish (Optional):**
   - For a delightful crispiness on top, you can broil the salmon for an additional 2-3 minutes. Keep a close eye to prevent burning.

8. **Serve and Garnish:**
   - Plate the Baked Salmon with Lemon and Herbs, garnishing with additional fresh herbs and lemon wedges for a burst of freshness.

9. **Pairing Suggestions:**
   - Serve this delightful baked salmon alongside a bed of quinoa, steamed vegetables, or a refreshing salad to create a well-balanced and satisfying meal.

10. **Enjoy the Culinary Delight:**
   - Revel in the succulence of the Baked Salmon with Lemon and Herbs, savoring each bite that captures the essence of fresh ingredients and culinary finesse.

This dish for baked salmon with herbs and lemon is a tribute to the skill of cooking with simplicity. With the zesty tones of lemon and the fragrant touch of herbs, it enhances the salmon's inherent flavours without taking away from them. This recipe is the epitome of what happens when simple cooking methods are combined with high-quality ingredients, making it ideal for both special occasions and weeknight dinners.

6.2 Turkey and Vegetable Stir-Fry

With this simple and healthy recipe that combines a variety of vibrant veggies with the lean deliciousness of turkey, you can turn your weekday meal into a gourmet experience. This stir-fry is a great addition to your arsenal of quick and delectable dinners since it not only guarantees a flavorful explosion but also offers a balanced serving of proteins and nutrients.

Ingredients:

- 1 pound ground turkey
- 2 tablespoons soy sauce
- 1 tablespoon oyster sauce
- 1 tablespoon hoisin sauce
- 2 tablespoons vegetable oil
- 2 cloves garlic, minced
- 1 tablespoon ginger, grated
- 1 red bell pepper, sliced
- 1 yellow bell pepper, sliced
- 1 cup broccoli florets
- 1 medium carrot, julienned
- 1 cup snap peas, ends trimmed
- Green onions for garnish
- Sesame seeds for garnish
- Cooked rice or noodles for serving

Instructions:

1. **Prepare the Sauce:**
   - Mix the hoisin sauce, oyster sauce, and soy sauce in a small bowl. This produces a thick, savoury sauce that is perfect for coating the turkey and veggies.

2. **Brown the Turkey:**
   - Heat the vegetable oil in a wok or big pan over medium-high heat. Using a spatula, break the ground turkey into crumbles while it cooks until it becomes brown.

3. **Add Aromatics:**
   - Add the grated ginger and minced garlic, stirring and sautéing until aromatic. The dish gains warmth and depth from these aromatics.

4. **Add Vegetables:**
   - Toss in the wok with the sliced red and yellow bell peppers, broccoli florets, julienned carrot, and snap peas. Stir-fry the veggies for three to four minutes, or until they are crisp-tender but not overdone.

6. **Garnish and Season:**

   - Add some chopped green onions and sesame seeds to the stir-fry to give it some texture. If needed, adjust the seasoning.

7. **Serve Over Rice or Noodles:**

   - Place a bed of cooked rice or noodles on which to place the Turkey and Vegetable Stir-Fry. The sauce is wonderful and will be absorbed by the soft grains or noodles.

8. **Savour Your Tasty Creation:**

   - Indulge in this colourful and healthful stir-fry and relish the harmony of flavorful sauces, crisp veggies, and soft turkey.

9. **Tailor to Your Taste:**

   - You are welcome to add more veggies to the stir-fry, such as baby corn, water chestnuts or mushrooms. A little amount of chilli sauce can also be used to change the degree of spiciness.

This stir-fried turkey and vegetable dish is a celebration of the flavorful and nutrient-dense balance that can be reached when lean protein and vibrant vegetables are combined, as well as a monument to how simple stir-frying can be. This dish demonstrates that a hearty and savoury supper can be both pleasurable and easily prepared, going from wok to plate in a matter of minutes.

6.3 Lentil and Vegetable Stew

Savour the comforting warmth and sustenance of a handmade lentil and vegetable stew, a hearty mélange that blends a bounty of colourful veggies with protein-rich lentils. This satisfying stew is a great addition to your repertoire of filling, nutrient-dense meals since it not only satisfies your hunger but also provides a symphony of flavours and vital nutrients.

Ingredients:

- 1 cup dry green or brown lentils, rinsed
- 2 tablespoons olive oil
- 1 onion, diced
- 2 carrots, chopped
- 2 celery stalks, chopped
- 3 cloves garlic, minced
- 1 teaspoon cumin
- 1 teaspoon paprika
- 1 teaspoon thyme
- 1 bay leaf
- 1 can (14 oz) diced tomatoes
- 4 cups vegetable broth
- 2 cups water
- Salt and pepper to taste
- Fresh parsley for garnish

Instructions:

1. **Rinse Lentils:**
   - First, give the dried lentils a quick rinse in cold water. This cleans them of any contaminants and gets them ready for cooking.

2. **Sauté Aromatics:**

- Place a big saucepan over medium heat with olive oil. Diced onions, chopped celery, and carrots should be sautéed until tender. When aromatic, add the minced garlic and continue to sauté.

3. **Add Spices:**

- Give the aromatic veggies a dash of cumin, paprika, thyme, and bay leaf. In order to unleash their flavours, stir the spices into the mixture.

4. **Add Lentils and Tomatoes:**

- Add diced tomatoes to the saucepan after adding the washed lentils. Mix everything together, being sure to cover the lentils well in the tasty sauce.

5. **Add Broth and Water:**

- Fill the saucepan with vegetable broth and water, then slowly bring the mixture to a boil. Reduce the heat to simmer and cover the pot.

6. **Simmer Until Lentils Are Tender:**
   - Simmer the stew for twenty to thirty minutes, or until the lentils are soft. Stir from time to time to avoid sticking.

7. **Season to Taste:**
   - Add salt and pepper to taste while seasoning the lentil and vegetable stew. Tailor the seasoning to your personal taste.

8. **Garnish and Serve:**
   - Spoon the filling stew into bowls, adding a finishing touch of fresh parsley for colour and freshness.

9. **Serve with Crusty Bread:**
   - For a genuinely filling supper, try this hearty lentil and vegetable stew by itself or with a slice of crusty bread.

10. **Store and Reheat:**
    - Put any leftovers in the fridge in an airtight container. When warmed, the flavours frequently intensify and become even more mouthwatering.

This Lentil and Vegetable Stew not only warms your soul with its comforting essence but also nourishes your body with a powerhouse of nutrients from lentils and a variety of vegetables. As each spoonful delivers a harmonious blend of flavors, you'll appreciate the simplicity and heartiness of this nutritious bowl of goodness.

CHAPTER SEVEN
HEALTHY DESSERTS FOR COGNITIVE WELLNESS

7.1 Berry and Yogurt Popsicles

Enjoy a tasty and nutritious treat of homemade berry and yoghurt popsicles to beat the summer heat. The natural sweetness of berries and the creamy deliciousness of yoghurt come together in this easy and colourful delight to create a frozen masterpiece that will cool you down and satisfy your sweet tooth with a blast of fruity freshness.

Ingredients:

- 1 cup mixed berries (strawberries, blueberries, raspberries)
- 2 cups Greek yogurt
- 1/4 cup honey or maple syrup (adjust to taste)
- 1 teaspoon vanilla extract
- Popsicle molds
- Popsicle sticks

Instructions:

1. **Prepare the Berry Mix:**
   - If used, wash and shell the strawberries. Blend the mixed berries in a blender until they are smooth. Leave some berry bits for texture if you like your texture chunkier.

2. **Sweeten and Flavour the Yoghurt:**
   - Combine Greek yoghurt, vanilla extract, and honey or maple syrup in a bowl. The tartness of the berries will go well with this yoghurt that has been sweetened.

3. **Layer the Popsicles:**
   - Spoon a tiny bit of the berry puree into each mould, then top it with a layer of yoghurt that has been sweetened.
   - Continue until all of the moulds are filled, producing an eye-catching striped look.

4. **Swirl for a Marbled Look:**
   - Gently swirl the layers together with a popsicle stick or skewer to create a marbled look. This adds a touch of artistry to your popsicles.

5. **Insert Popsicle Sticks:**
   - Make sure the popsicle sticks are centred in each popsicle before inserting them into the moulds. To hold the sticks in place, the yoghurt and berry mixture will freeze around them.

6. **Freeze Until Solid:**
   - Freeze the popsicles in the freezer for four to six hours, or until they solidify. For optimal results, freezing overnight is recommended.

7. **Unmold and Enjoy:**
   - To release the popsicles from the moulds once they have completely frozen, briefly submerge them in warm water. Pull them out gently and savour the cool delight.

8. **Optional Extras:**
   - For an added layer of decadence, roll the completed popsicles in chopped almonds, shredded coconut, or even a drizzle of melted dark chocolate.

9. **Share the Joy:**
   - Share these homemade Berry and Yogurt Popsicles with friends and family, spreading the joy of a cool and delightful summer treat.

10. **Experiment with Variations:**
   - Get creative by experimenting with different berries, adding citrus zest, or incorporating a handful of granola for a crunchy surprise.

These Berry and Yogurt Popsicles are not just frozen delights; they are a celebration of summer's bounty, bringing together the lusciousness of berries and the creaminess of yogurt in a convenient and refreshing form. With every lick, savor the essence of summer encapsulated in this homemade frozen treat.

7.2 Baked Apple Slices with Cinnamon

Simple Baked Apple Slices, caressed by a hint of aromatic cinnamon, turn crisp apples into a warm and comfortable delicacy. This simple dish offers a delicious balance of natural sweetness and spice, as well as a tantalising scent that fills your kitchen. These baked apple slices are a tribute to the magic that occurs when fresh food meets the warmth of your oven. They're ideal for a cosy evening or as a nutritious dessert alternative.

Ingredients:
- 4-5 medium-sized apples (a sweet variety like Honeycrisp or Fuji works well)
- 2 tablespoons melted butter or coconut oil
- 2 tablespoons brown sugar or maple syrup
- 1 teaspoon ground cinnamon
- 1/4 teaspoon nutmeg (optional)
- A pinch of salt

Instructions:

1. **Preheat the Oven:**
- Preheat your oven to 375°F (190°C). This ensures a gentle and even bake for the apple slices.

2. **Prepare the Apples:**
   - Peel (if desired) and core the apples after washing. To ensure consistent baking, cut them into thin, uniform pieces.

3. **Apply Melted Butter:**
   - Evenly cover the apple slices in melted butter or coconut oil by tossing them in a big basin. This enhances the flavour and makes the cinnamon mixture stick to the slices better.

4. Make the Cinnamon Sugar Blend:
   - In a small bowl, combine the ground cinnamon, nutmeg (if using), brown sugar or maple syrup, and a little amount of salt. This fragrant mixture gives the apples a covering that is both sweet and spicy.

5. **Coat Apple Slices:**
   - Generously coat each apple slice by sprinkling it with the cinnamon sugar mixture. To uniformly spread the ingredients, lightly toss the pieces.

6. **Arrange on Baking Sheet:**
   - Use parchment paper to line a baking sheet. To ensure consistent baking, place the coated apple slices in a single layer without packing them too tightly.

7. **Bake Until Tender:**
   - Bake the apple slices in the preheated oven for 20 to 25 minutes, or until they are soft and have a hint of colour. Halfway through, stir to ensure even baking.

8. **Allow to Cool Slightly and Serve:**
   - Before serving, let the baked apple slices cool slightly. The smell of cinnamon mixed with the warmth of cooked apples makes for a lovely sensory experience.

9. **Serve with Toppings (Optional):**
   - To add texture, you might serve the baked apple slices with a scoop of ice cream, a dollop of vanilla yoghurt, or a sprinkling of chopped nuts.

10. **Enjoy the Sweet Comfort:**
    - Relish in the sweet comfort of Baked Apple Slices with Cinnamon, savoring each bite that encapsulates the essence of

fall and the simple joy of a homemade dessert.

These Baked Apple Slices with Cinnamon are a testament to the beauty of uncomplicated desserts. With just a handful of ingredients, you can transform ordinary apples into a warm, spiced indulgence that brings the cozy flavors of fall to your table. Enjoy the natural sweetness, warmth, and fragrance of this delightful treat.

7.3 Dark Chocolate Avocado Mousse

Dark Chocolate Avocado Mousse is a rich, velvety dessert that combines the deliciousness of dark chocolate with the creaminess of avocados, taking you on a voyage of guilt-free delight. This rich mousse adds a healthy twist by using nutrient-dense avocados in addition to satisfying your sweet taste. Prepare to up your dessert game with this easy yet opulent dish.

Ingredients:

- 2 ripe avocados, peeled and pitted
- 1/2 cup dark chocolate chips or chopped dark chocolate (70% cocoa or higher).
- 1/4 cup unsweetened cocoa powder
- 1/4 cup maple syrup or agave nectar
- 1 teaspoon vanilla extract
- A pinch of salt
- Fresh berries or mint leaves for garnish (optional)

Instructions:

1. **Melt Dark Chocolate:**
   - To start, melt chopped or chipped dark chocolate. You may melt it in the microwave in small bursts or using a double boiler. Once smooth, remove and allow to cool slightly.

2. **Blend Avocados:**
   - Put ripe avocados, chocolate powder, vanilla extract, maple syrup or agave nectar, and a dash of salt in a food processor or blender. Blend until the mixture is fully blended and creamy.

3. **Add Melted Chocolate:**
   - Stir the dark chocolate into the avocado mixture after it has melted. Repeatedly blend until all of the chocolate is combined, resulting in a smooth and decadent mousse.

4. **Taste and Adjust Sweetness:**
   - If additional maple syrup or agave nectar is required, taste the mousse and adjust the sweetness. Blend just long enough to mix.

5. **Chill the Mousse:**
   - Spoon the Dark Chocolate Avocado Mousse into dishes or glasses for serving. To let the flavours combine and the mousse set, chill in the fridge for at least two hours.

6. **Garnish and Serve:**
   - To add a pop of colour and freshness, top the mousse with fresh berries or mint leaves just before serving. Although optional, this step brings a nice touch.

7. **Savour the Smooth Joy:**
   - Savour the rich flavour and velvety texture of Dark Chocolate Avocado Mousse. Every bite celebrates the union of nutritious components and opulent appeal.

8. **Play Around with the Toppings:**
   - Add some flare to your dish by adding a dusting of cocoa powder, a drizzle of coconut cream, or a sprinkling of chopped nuts.

9. **Share the Delight:**
   - Share this guilt-free indulgence with friends and family, surprising them with the revelation that avocados can transform into a silky, chocolatey delight.

10. **Appreciate the Nutrient Boost:**
   - As you savor each spoonful, appreciate the nutrient boost from avocados, providing healthy fats, fiber, and a dose of vitamins to this luxurious dessert.

This Dark Chocolate Avocado Mousse is not just a dessert; it's a testament to the magic of combining wholesome ingredients to create a treat that satisfies both your sweet cravings and your desire for nutrient-dense indulgence. Enjoy the silky richness and savor the decadent flavors guilt-free.

CHAPTER EIGHT
BEVERAGES THAT NOURISH THE BRAIN

8.1 Green Tea with Mint

The revitalising mix of Green Tea with Mint will elevate your tea-drinking experience. It combines the earthy notes of green tea with the cold, refreshing aroma of mint in a harmonic combination. In addition to providing a relaxing diversion, this wonderful beverage combines the digestive qualities of mint with the antioxidant benefits of green tea. Prepare to go on a peaceful and restorative trip with this straightforward but energising tea.

Ingredients:

- 1 green tea bag or 1 teaspoon loose green tea leaves
- Fresh mint leaves (about 4-6 leaves)
- 1 teaspoon honey or sweetener of choice (optional)
- Boiling water

Instructions:

1. **Select Quality Green Tea:**
   - Start by selecting loose green tea leaves or a premium green tea bag. Select a type of green tea that you enjoy drinking, such sencha, matcha, or jasmine.

2. **Boil Water:**
   - Heat the water until it boils. Use fresh, filtered water for the finest flavour.

3. **Brew Green Tea:**
   - Fill a teapot or cup with loose leaves or a green tea bag. After adding boiling water to the tea, let it steep for two to three minutes.
   - Depending on the strength you want, adjust the steeping time.

4. **Add Fresh Mint Leaves:**
   - Gently crush the fresh mint leaves with your fingertips to release their oils and scent while the green tea steeps. In the mug or teapot, add the mint leaves.

5. **Sweeten if Desired:**
   - Add honey or your favourite sweetener to the green tea if you'd like a little sweetness. For it to dissolve, give it a good stir.

6. **Strain or Remove Tea Bag:**
   - You can choose to strain away the loose leaves or remove the tea bag once the green tea has steeped to your preferred consistency. In doing so, you may avoid oversteeping and preserve the delicate flavour of the tea.

7. **Present and Savour:**
   - Fill your preferred cup with the infused green tea with mint. Earthy green tea and energising mint combine to provide a flavour profile that is both refreshing and well-balanced.

8. **Garnish with Mint (Optional):**
   - Add a sprig of fresh mint to your tea to add a little more elegance. This amplifies the scent of mint and improves the appearance as well.

9. **Sip and Relax:**
   - Savor each sip of Green Tea with Mint, allowing the delicate dance of flavors to soothe your senses and provide a moment of relaxation.

10. **Experiment with Variations:**
   - Feel free to experiment with variations, such as adding a splash of lemon juice or adjusting the mint quantity to suit your taste preferences.

This Green Tea with Mint isn't just a beverage; it's a ritual that combines the ancient elegance of green tea with the revitalizing touch of fresh mint. Whether enjoyed as a morning pick-me-up or an afternoon respite, this tea promises a refreshing journey for your taste buds and a tranquil moment for your soul.

8.2 Berry and Spinach Smoothie

Smoothies that mix the nutrient-rich strength of spinach with the sweet appeal of berries are a great way to invigorate your day. Try the Berry and Spinach Smoothie. This tasty smoothie is a great option for a nutritious and delectable drink since it tantalises your taste buds while providing a boost of fibre, vitamins, and antioxidants.

Ingredients:
- 1 cup mixed berries (strawberries, blueberries, raspberries)
- 1 cup fresh spinach leaves
- 1 banana, peeled
- 1/2 cup Greek yogurt
- 1 tablespoon chia seeds (optional)
- 1 cup unsweetened almond milk or your preferred liquid
- Ice cubes (optional)

Instructions:
1. **Gather Fresh Ingredients:**
   - Gather fresh mixed berries, spinach, ripe banana, Greek yoghurt, unsweetened almond milk, and chia seeds (if using).

2. **Prepare the Ingredients:**
   - Give the spinach and berries a good wash. To make mixing easier, peel and chop the banana.
3. **Load the Blender:**
   - Fill a blender with the mixed berries, banana pieces, fresh spinach leaves, Greek yoghurt, and chia seeds, if using.
4. **Add Liquid and Ice:**
   - To ensure a smooth blending process, add the unsweetened almond milk. Include a few ice cubes as well if you like your smoothie to be cooler.
5. **Blend Until Smooth:**
   - Use a high-speed blender to blend the ingredients together until the sauce is creamy and smooth.
   - If needed, take a moment to scrape down the blender's sides.
6. **Check Consistency and Adjust:**
   - Verify how consistent the smoothie is. Add extra almond milk if it's too thick, and more frozen berries or ice cubes if it's too thin.

7. **Taste and Adjust Sweetness:**
   - If necessary, adjust the sweetness of the smoothie after tasting it.
   - A teaspoon of honey or maple syrup might be added, depending on how sweet the berries are.

8. **Pour and Serve:**
   - Fill a glass with the delicious Berry and Spinach Smoothie.
   - This smoothie is visually beautiful and delicious at the same time because of its brilliant colour and inviting scent.

9. **Garnish (Optional):**
   - Add some whole berries or chia seeds to your smoothie as a finishing touch. This gives it a fun visual flare and delicious crunch.

10. **Sip and Rejoice in Health:**
    - Sip on your Berry and Spinach Smoothie, relishing the fusion of sweet berries, the earthy goodness of spinach, and the creamy texture from Greek yogurt. Each sip is a celebration of health and vitality.

This Berry and Spinach Smoothie is not merely a beverage; it's a celebration of the bountiful nutrients nature provides. Packed with vitamins, antioxidants, and a refreshing flavor profile, this smoothie is a delicious and wholesome way to nourish your body and invigorate your senses.

8.3 Coconut Water with a Splash of Citrus

With the revitalising combination of Coconut Water with a Splash of Citrus, you may transport yourself to a tropical paradise. This hydrating elixir blends the naturally sweet taste of coconut water with the zesty energy of citrus fruits. This revitalising drink is ideal for a warm day since it not only satisfies your thirst but also gives you a boost of vitamins, minerals, and electrolytes.

Ingredients:
- 1 cup fresh coconut water
- 1/2 lime or lemon, juiced
- 1 tablespoon orange juice
- Ice cubes
- Mint leaves for garnish (optional)

Instructions:

1. **Extract Fresh Coconut Water:**
   - Begin by extracting fresh coconut water. If using a young coconut, carefully open it and collect the water. Alternatively, use store-bought coconut water without added sugars.

2. **Prepare Citrus Juices:**
   - Juice half a lime or lemon to add a zesty kick to the coconut water. Additionally, squeeze the juice from an orange for a touch of sweetness.

3. **Combine Coconut Water and Citrus Juices:**
   - In a glass, combine the fresh coconut water with the lime or lemon juice and orange juice. The combination of these citrus flavors enhances the natural sweetness of the coconut water.

4. **Add Ice Cubes:**
   - Drop a few ice cubes into the glass to chill the beverage and create a refreshing contrast to the tropical flavors.

5. **Stir Well:**
   - Stir the Coconut Water with a Splash of Citrus thoroughly to ensure the citrus juices are evenly distributed, providing a harmonious blend of sweet and tangy notes.

6. **Garnish with Mint (Optional):**
   - For an extra touch of freshness, garnish your tropical refresher with a few mint leaves. The aromatic essence of mint complements the citrus and coconut flavors.

7. **Serve Chilled:**
   - Present your Coconut Water with a Splash of Citrus chilled and ready to be enjoyed. The visual appeal of the clear liquid with citrus accents is as enticing as its taste.

8. **Sip and Rehydrate:**
   - Sip on this tropical concoction, reveling in the hydrating properties of coconut water while enjoying the burst of citrusy zest. The drink not only quenches your thirst

but also provides a replenishing dose of electrolytes.

9. **Experiment with Variations:**
   - Feel free to experiment with variations, such as adding a splash of pineapple juice, a hint of ginger, or even a sprinkle of sea salt for a nuanced flavor profile.

10. **Relax and Enjoy the Tropical Escape:**
   - Whether lounging by the pool or seeking a mid-afternoon pick-me-up, Coconut Water with a Splash of Citrus offers a tropical escape in every sip. Enjoy the refreshing simplicity and tropical allure of this hydrating elixir.

This Coconut Water with a Splash of Citrus not only hydrates and refreshes but also transports you to a beachside paradise with its tropical fusion of coconut sweetness and citrus vibrancy. Embrace the simplicity of this revitalizing drink as you savor the natural flavors of the tropics in every sip.

CHAPTER NINE
TIPS FOR INCORPORATING BRAIN-BOOSTING FOODS

9.1 Meal Planning Strategies

Meal planning is an effective strategy that not only makes meal preparation easier but also lowers stress, promotes cost savings, and results in healthier eating habits. To help you organise your meals more efficiently and enjoy cooking more, consider the following:

1. **Weekly Meal Planning:**
   - Set aside a particular day of the week to organise your meals. Make a meal plan based on the foods you currently have by taking stock of your pantry, refrigerator, and freezer.

2. **Create a Menu:**
   - List a range of meals that should be served on a monthly or biweekly basis. A good mix of fruits, grains, vegetables, and proteins should be included. This gives

your meals organisation and promotes a range of nutrients.

3. **Consider Dietary Goals:**

   - Whether your objective is to lose weight, increase muscle, or meet a certain dietary need, make sure your meal plan reflects these objectives. Select recipes that help you achieve your goals.

4. **Batch Cooking:**

   - Save time by preparing ingredients in batches. Make a lot of staple foods like grains, meats, and sauces so you can eat them for several meals a week.

5. **Theme Nights:**

   - Designate particular nights, such Taco Tuesday, Stir-Fry Friday, or Meatless Monday. This makes choosing meals easier and gives your meals more diversity.

6. **Adaptability with Leftovers:**

   - See leftovers as a useful resource. Intentionally overcook some food to provide easy and quick dinners the following day or later in the week.

7. **Utilize Seasonal Produce:**
   - Toss recipes with seasonal produce and fruits in mind. They bring diversity to your diet, are frequently cheaper and fresher.

8. **Grocery List Mastery:**
   - Make an extensive grocery list based on your weekly schedule. Sort things by category to make your shopping trip go more quickly and reduce the likelihood that you will forget something.

9. **Prepare Ahead of Time:**
   - Set some time to prepare meals. Prepare grains ahead of time, wash and slice veggies, or marinade meats. During hectic workdays, preparing meals is accelerated when items are prepared in advance.

10. **Remain Inspired:**
    - As a source of inspiration, maintain a compilation of your best recipes, culinary blogs, or cookbooks. You may avoid culinary boredom and keep your meals interesting by experimenting with different dishes.

11. **Mindful Budgeting:**
   - Make food plans that are within your means. Cost reductions can be achieved by selecting seasonal food, buying in bulk, and adding reasonably priced proteins.

12. **Technology Support:**
   - Make use of applications or internet resources for meal planning that provide recipe recommendations, the ability to create shopping lists, and nutritional data. The planning process may be streamlined with these tools.

13. **Pay Attention to Your Schedule:**
   - Take it into account while organising your meals. Choose quick and simple meals for hectic days and save more complex ones for days when you have more time.

14. **Assess and Modify:**
   - Evaluate your food planning techniques on a regular basis. Determine what was successful and what needed improvement. Modify your strategy to better fit your changing tastes and demands.

By implementing these meal planning strategies, you can transform your approach to cooking, making it more efficient, enjoyable, and aligned with your health and lifestyle goals. Meal planning not only saves time but also contributes to a more mindful and intentional approach to nourishing yourself and your loved ones.

9.2 Grocery Shopping for Brain Health

The key to grocery shopping for brain health is to choose nutrient-dense foods that promote mental health in general and cognitive function in particular. During your next grocery shop, use this tips to help you make decisions that will benefit your brain:

1. **Fatty Fish:** When making your grocery list, be sure to include fatty fish like salmon, trout, and sardines. These are abundant in omega-3 fatty acids, which are believed to enhance cognitive function and are vital for the health of the brain.

2. **Leafy Greens:** Eat a lot of Swiss chard, spinach and kale, among other leafy greens. These leafy greens, which are abundant in vitamins, minerals, and antioxidants, support brain function and guard against cognitive ageing.

3. **Berries:** Antioxidants and flavonoids abound in berries, particularly blueberries. There is evidence linking these chemicals to enhanced cognitive function and memory.

4. **Nuts and Seeds:** Spread out your selection of nuts and seeds, including almonds, walnuts, chia seeds, and flaxseeds. They are also rich in antioxidants, vitamin E, and omega-3 fatty acids, all of which are beneficial to brain function.

5. **Whole Grains:** Go for whole grains such as oats, brown rice, and quinoa. These offer a consistent delivery of glucose, the brain's main energy source.

6. **Avocado:** Packed with monounsaturated fats, avocados support normal blood circulation. Increased blood flow can improve cognitive performance and maintain a healthy brain.

7. **Broccoli:** Vitamin K, which is necessary for the formation of sphingolipids—a type of fat that is densely packed into brain cells, and antioxidants are abundant in broccoli.

8. **Eggs:** Choline is one of the several nutrients that are abundant in eggs. Acetylcholine, a neurotransmitter crucial for mood and memory control, is derived from choline.

9. **Turmeric:** Add some turmeric to your assortment of spices. The main ingredient in turmeric, curcumin, has antioxidant and anti-inflammatory properties that may improve brain function.

10. **Dark Chocolate:** Treat yourself to some rich, dark chocolate. Flavonoids, antioxidants, and caffeine found in dark chocolate may improve mood and memory.

11. **Oranges and other Citrus Fruits:** Vitamin C, which is essential for avoiding mental deterioration, is abundant in citrus fruits like oranges. Additionally, they include antioxidants, which may shield the brain.

12. **Pumpkin Seeds:** Rich in antioxidants, magnesium, iron, zinc, and copper, pumpkin seeds are a fantastic source of these nutrients. These minerals play a role in brain function and overall mental well-being.

13. **Green Tea:** Put green tea on your list of things to buy. Caffeine and L-theanine, which are found in green tea, may work in concert to enhance mood and cognitive function.

14. **Beets:** Nitrates found in beets may enhance blood flow to the brain, hence enhancing cognitive performance. They also possess anti-inflammatory and antioxidant qualities.

15. **Low-Fat Dairy:** Consume dairy products with less fat, such as milk and yoghurt. They have a high vitamin D content, which has been linked to a lower incidence of cognitive deterioration.

Putting these brain-boosting items at the top of your grocery list can improve general health and wellbeing as well as cognitive performance. Mix and match these ingredients to make a variety of wholesome meals that feed your body and mind.

9.3 Cooking Techniques to Retain Nutrients

To guarantee that you get the most out of the vitamins, minerals, and other vital elements, food's nutritional value must be preserved throughout cooking. The following cooking methods will help you preserve the nutritious value of your food:

1. **Steaming:** Steaming reduces nutritional loss and is a gentle cooking method. It includes cooking food using steam to retain colour and nutrition. You can steam vegetables, seafood, and cereals to keep them nutritious.

2. **Microwaving:** This rapid and effective technique can help keep food's nutrients intact. It minimises nutritional deterioration and cuts down on cooking time by producing heat inside the meal.

3. **Sautéing:** Food is rapidly cooked in a tiny amount of oil over medium to high heat while sautéing. Because this method cooks food quickly, nutrients are retained, especially when high-quality oils like olive oil are used.

4. **Blanching:** Blanching is the process of quickly submerging food in boiling water and then chilling it down in icy water. This method softens veggies just a bit while preserving their rich colour and nutrition.

5. **Grilling and broiling:** These high-heat cooking techniques, particularly for meats, help preserve nutrients. When grilling, extra fat falls off and cooking times are often lower than with other cooking techniques.

6. **Slow Cooking:** Maintaining nutritional levels can be achieved by slow cooking for a longer period of time at lower temperatures. This method is particularly suitable for tougher cuts of meat and legumes.

7. **Pressure Cooking:** Pressure cooking reduces cooking time and helps retain water-soluble vitamins. It's especially beneficial for legumes and grains, preserving their nutritional content.

8. **Raw or Lightly Cooked:** Eating raw or lightly cooked vegetables and fruits ensures that their nutrients remain intact. Consider incorporating salads, smoothies, and raw snacks into your diet.

9. **Using Cooking Liquids:** Cooking liquids, such broth or water used to boil vegetables, should be saved and utilised again. You may stop nutritional loss by adding these liquids to stews, soups, and sauces.

10. **Steer clear of overcooking:** This might cause nutrients to be lost. When preparing vegetables in particular, pay attention to the prescribed cooking periods and steer clear of too high heat.

11. **Minimise Peeling:** Try to keep fruit and vegetable skins on them since they frequently contain important fibre and minerals.

12. **Cooking in Bulk:** Take into account batch cooking while making huge amounts of food. By doing this, food is exposed to less heat for a longer period of time, retaining more nutrients.

13. **Using Minimal Water:** Use the least quantity of water required for simmering or boiling. This reduces the leaching of water-soluble vitamins into the cooking liquid.

14. **Adding Acidic Ingredients:** Incorporate acidic ingredients like citrus juice or vinegar into your recipes. Acid can help preserve the color and nutritional content of certain fruits and vegetables.

By incorporating these cooking techniques into your meal preparation, you can maximize the retention of nutrients in your food, ensuring that you receive the full range of health benefits from the ingredients you choose.

CONCLUSION

Embracing a Brain-Healthy Lifestyle

Adopting a brain-healthy lifestyle is essential for seniors to maintain memory, cognitive function, and general mental wellness. In order to promote elders' mental health, keep the following points in mind:

1. **Nutrient-Rich Diet:** Make eating a variety of fruits, vegetables, whole grains, lean meats, and healthy fats a top priority. Your diet should also be balanced and rich in nutrients. The health of the brain is influenced by vitamins, antioxidants, and omega-3 fatty acids.

2. **Maintain Proper Hydration:** Drinking enough water is crucial for good health in general, including mental clarity. Seniors should be encouraged to sip on enough water throughout the day.

3. **Consistent Exercise:** Take part in consistent physical exercise. Exercise boosts general cognitive function, lowers the risk of chronic illnesses, and increases blood flow to the brain. Walking, swimming, and mild aerobics are a few examples of helpful activities.

4. **Mental Stimulation:** Mental stimulus helps to maintain mental activity. Reading, solving puzzles, playing board games, picking up new skills, and learning new things all support cognitive function and may lower the risk of cognitive decline.

5. **Proper Sleep:** Make sure elderly people receive adequate restorative sleep. For the brain to function properly and to consolidate memories, good sleep is essential. Create a cosy sleeping environment and stick to a regular sleep schedule.

6. **Social Engagement:** Promote engagement and social relationships. Keeping up relationships with friends, family, and the community supports emotional health and reduces feelings of loneliness.

7. **Stress Management:** Instruct students in stress-reduction methods including deep breathing exercises, mindfulness, and meditation. The long-term effects of chronic stress on cognitive performance make it critical to develop constructive coping strategies.

8. **Regular Health Check-ups:** Make time for routine checkups with your doctor to monitor and treat diseases including high blood pressure, diabetes, and high cholesterol. When left unchecked, these disorders can exacerbate cognitive deterioration.

9. **Restrict Alcohol and Quit Smoking:** Give elders advice on how to reduce their alcohol intake and, if necessary, stop smoking. An higher risk of cognitive deterioration has been associated with both drinking and smoking.

10. **Medication Management:** Make sure that medications are properly managed. Seniors should take their prescriptions as directed, and they should talk to medical experts about any adverse effects or concerns.

11. **Stick to a Schedule:** Create a daily schedule that consists of regular activities, food, and exercise. A regimented schedule gives one a feeling of security and has a good effect on mental health.

12. **Interests and Hobbies:** Motivate elders to engage in interests and hobbies. Engaging in meaningful and enjoyable pursuits contributes to a sense of purpose and happiness.

13. **Brain-Healthy Foods:** Consume foods high in omega-3 fatty acids, blueberries, dark leafy greens, nuts, and seeds, as well as other brain-healthy nutrients. Nutrients in these diets promote cognitive function.

14. **Schedule Regular Screenings:** Make time for routine hearing and vision exams. Sustaining sensory health is critical to safety and general cognitive function.

15. **Adaptation and Support:** Acknowledge any changes in cognition and offer assistance. Seniors who want to keep their independence might benefit from emotional support, memory aids, and living space adaptations.

Seniors may actively support the maintenance of cognitive function, foster mental wellness, and lead satisfying, healthy lives as they age by adopting certain lifestyle practises. It's critical to customise these suggestions to each person's requirements and tastes while consulting medical specialists for advice.